Nutrition, Your Way

Nutrition, Your Way

*Josh Bryant, Adam benShea,
and Stefan de Kort*

Nutrition, Your Way

JoshStrength, LLC and Adam benShea

Copyright © 2018

All rights reserved, including file sharing and the right to reproduce this work, in whole or any part, in any form. All inquiries must be directed to Josh Bryant and Adam benShea and have approval from both authors.

Table of Contents

Introduction vii

Step 1: Calories 1

Step 2: Macros 10

Step 3: Food Selection 17

Step 4: Meal Frequency 23

Step 5: Nutrient Timing 26

Step 6: Hydration 32

Step 7: Diet Breaks and Refeeds 35

Step 8: Supplements 41

Closing Thoughts 47

References 49

Introduction

Imprisonment takes many different forms.

With that statement, profound in its simplicity and sincerity, the *Jailhouse Strong* movement started.

Our first book, and the growing list of titles after it, offered a means to break free from your particular form of imprisonment. Specifically, we offered the solution of strength. It is with strength that you are able to endure your predicament and improve your reality. It is with strength that you display your ability to make the most of what you have and where you are.

We helped our readers cultivate not just physical strength, but mental and emotional strength as well. We did this with books on old-school physical culture, interval training, and goal setting.

Many got stronger, but many still felt trapped, or imprisoned, inside of their own body. This is not a good feeling. We responded with our runaway bestseller, *Keto Built*.

This book changed lives and bodies. As a consequence of *Keto Built*, backs are even broader, waists are leaner, and people are healthier. The folks who do well with Keto thrive with it. The issue, for different reasons, is that not everybody performs well on Keto.

We are grateful that we were able to help so many, and we want to help even more folks. To do that, we created this book as a means to offer an outline and nutritional program that can be customized to the specific needs of just about anyone.

If you follow *Jailhouse Strong* on Instagram and regularly watch our videos on the *Jailhouse Strong* YouTube channel, you have heard us discuss the concept of the individual over the institution. This means that we believe in appealing to the intuition of the individual over blindly following conventional allegiance to the large institution. With commitment to that philosophy, we provide this book as an individualized guidebook.

The way of the individual may be best summed up with the wisdom of "Ol' Blue Eyes," Frank Sinatra. A cult hero from a bygone era, Sinatra was admired for his voice and stage presence. But in addition to that, Mafia bosses and creative artists alike respected Sinatra because he bucked the system, broke the mold, and did it "his way."

He lived his own life.

So, in the tradition of "Ol' Blue Eyes" himself, you can do it "your way."

In this book, we provide the information, the research, and the means for application. You decide what works best for you, your lifestyle, and your nutritional goals.

With that in mind, this could be *your* most potent nutrition guide.

Why?

Two reasons.

First, this book is fluff-free. Every concept is extremely actionable. We provide you with a step-by-step approach to set up your customized nutrition plan based on your personal situation, needs, and preferences. We'll do this by first discovering the fundamentals and nuances of effective dieting—ranging from calorie counting to supplements and everything in between—and then showing you how to put everything into action, starting today!

Our objective is to help you build a nutrition plan that works optimally and specifically for you. So whether you're a student, a stay-at-home dad, or a jet-setting business professional who's always on the go, your diet will fit your needs and lifestyle.

Second, everything found in this book is based on scientific research (and, for those bean counters, we've cited every study so that you can easily review the data yourself). The concepts you're about to discover are based on proven principles and methods. In other words, this is not the regular bro-science that's running rampant in the world of health and fitness.

Now, before we dive in, one crucial note: This book is outlined in a step-by-step fashion, and each section builds on the previous one. So it's vital that you go through this resource in the presented order. The material is presented in a hierarchical fashion. The foundational information is described first, and the material to take your nutritional plan to the pinnacle of success is presented last.

Also, most chapters contain a few simple but important exercises. When you reach those, do them immediately because you'll need that info for the subsequent chapters. Got it? Great! Then settle in and study this book, because you don't want to miss this. Let's get started!

Step 1: Calories

Calories are the most important but most often neglected dieting fundamental. Here's how you can get this right.

Whether you're stepping out to play the field or setting foot on the field of play, there's one nutrition factor that most significantly influences your results. No, it's not meal frequency, glycemic index, or food selection (although those are important, as we'll discuss later). Calorie intake is what largely determines which direction the scale moves. In this section, you'll discover why calories are important, and how many of them you should consume for optimal results.

Calories: What Are They and Why Should You Care?

A calorie is a unit that measures energy, usually energy found in foods and beverages. The connection between caloric consumption and body weight is pretty straightforward. In fact, the research is evident on this one: If you want to lose, maintain, or gain weight, calories are the most crucial factor to get in check. It's simple. If you consume more calories than you burn, you'll gain weight. And if you consume fewer calories than you burn, you'll lose weight.[1-19]

Now like with almost every aspect of fitness and nutrition, there are so-called gurus (along with their "flock") who may claim that calories are obsolete. That's hogwash.

Regulating calorie balance is the factor around which all weight-loss diets are based, whether the promoters of the eating style admit it or not. All of these plans are designed to help you—whether consciously or unconsciously—consume fewer calories than you burn, and by doing so cause you to lose weight. (Yes, this includes Atkins, the

Paleo diet, the ketogenic diet, the Zone diet, the 5:2 diet, and so forth.) The same is true for weight-gain diets, but in the inverse. When you follow a proper mass-gaining plan, the number on your scale increases because you are consuming more calories than your body burns.

Want proof? Well, dozens of scientific studies show the validity of calorie balance.[1-18] For example, over the last decades, the lab coats in the research halls have done many "overfeeding studies." During these studies, participants are instructed to overeat, and then scientists measure how this impacts their weight and health. The result? Well, the participants aren't eager to wear swimsuits at their next condo complex pool party, because they packed on the pounds. All of these studies show that when people eat more calories than they burn, they gain weight.[18-25]

It's that simple.

The same holds true for losing weight—if you consume fewer calories than you burn, you'll lose weight. An interesting case study showing this to be true was done by Mark Haub, a professor of human nutrition at Kansas State University.[26] He carried excess pounds before the trial, so knowing the importance of calorie balance, he decided to do an experiment. For two months, he stuck with gas station foods such as Twinkies, Oreos, Doritos, and protein shakes while maintaining a daily caloric deficit of 800 calories. Now, in agreement with Professor Haub, we don't recommend you follow such a diet. But the results are amazing. In just two months he lost 27 pounds and reduced his body fat from 33.4 percent to 24.9 percent.

While that's not lean enough to hit the male revue stage, you're on your way to getting #chippendalesready.

The important lesson is this: Studies show that when people eat fewer calories than they burn, they lose weight.

It's that simple.

Determining Your Optimal Calorie Intake

It should be clear by now that calories play a crucial role for your physique, whether you want to gain, maintain, or lose weight.

But how many calories should you consume to reach your fitness goals? The following four-step formula provides the answer. Go through the calculations to discover your daily calorie needs based on your goals and situation.

Important note: The following section requires calculations. It's crucial that you do these because they form the foundation of your diet, and you'll need the results for the upcoming chapters. While we've done our best to make the calculations as easy and straightforward as possible, if you're having difficulty with the math, please use the links we've included (and remember your smartphone has a calculator). These will make it easier to go through the formulas.

First, calculate your BMR

Your basal metabolic rate—or BMR, for short—refers to how many calories you would burn in a day if you were to do no physical activities. Calculating this number is the first step in figuring out your ideal calorie intake. Do this by using the following formula:[27]

- BMR for men = (10 × weight in kg) + (6.25 × height in cm) − (5 × age in years) + 5
- BMR for women = (10 × weight in kg) + (6.25 × height in cm) − (5 × age in years) − 161

Examples:

The following are examples of a 26-year-old man who is 5'10" (178 cm) and weighs 176 pounds (80 kg) and a 38-year-old woman who is 5'4½" (164 cm) and 121 pounds (55 kg).

- BMR men: (10 × 80) + (6.25 × 178) − (5 × 26) + 5 = 1,788
- BMR women: (10 × 55) + (6.25 × 164) − (5 × 38) − 161 = 1,224

Secondly, adjust to activity level

Because physical activity influences calorie output, it's important to take this factor into consideration. We do this by using the activity multiplier below. It's simple. First, you select the activity level that best describes your current situation. Then you apply the multiplier to your BMR (the number that you calculated in the previous step).

- Sedentary (little or no exercise and a desk job) => BMR x 1.2
- Lightly active (light activity with light exercise or sports 1 to 3 days a week) => BMR x 1.375
- Moderately active (moderate activity with moderate exercise or sports 3 to 5 days a week) => BMR x 1.55
- Very active (much activity or hard exercise or sports 6 to 7 days a week) => BMR x 1.725
- Extremely active (hard daily exercise or activity and physical work) => BMR x 1.9

Example:
Let's say that your activity levels fall under the category "moderately active" and your BMR is 1,650 calories. In such a case, your calculation would look as follows:

1,650 x 1.55 = 2,558

Thirdly, modify toward your primary goal
Here's how:

- If your primary goal is losing body fat, subtract 500 calories.
- If your primary goal is gaining mass, add 300 calories.
- If you want to maintain your current body weight, don't change your previously calculated number.

Example:
The hypothetical moderately active person we considered in the previous step would start by consuming 2,858 calories to gain muscle (2,558 + 300 = 2,858) and 2,058 to lose body fat (2,558 – 500 = 2,058).

Fourthly, update according to your progress

While these calculations are generally very accurate, you may have to adjust your calorie intake as time progresses. One reason for this is that your body may adapt to your eating style. For example, if you reduce your calorie intake, your body tends to downregulate its metabolic rate to prevent you from losing more weight. Essentially, this is because your body believes that it is starving and a survival instinct kicks in to prevent starvation. That is, your body burns calories at a slower rate. For some people, such dieting-induced reductions in calorie output are severe. For others, they're minimal.

The same holds true for building muscle. When you consume more calories than you burn, your metabolism may increase to prevent excess weight gain. Now, once again, such increases in calorie output are severe for some people and minimal for others.

Remember, this is an individual approach to nutrition, so you'll need to make adjustments based on who you are and how you live.

In recognition that your body may adjust to changes in calorie intake, you might have to increase or decrease your energy consumption as time progresses. Here's how to figure out whether you should adjust your calorie intake:

First, make it a habit to step on the scale every morning. Do this upon awakening, and after using the restroom, but before consuming breakfast or drinking any liquids. Write down the number every day and then, at the end of the week, add them all up. Divide this number by seven to get your average weight for that week. (You can use the following free application to calculate your weekly average: **https://www.omnicalculator.com/math/average**.)

Second, calculate in percentages how much your body weight changes each week. You do this by using the following formula:

(old weight – new weight) / (old weight x 100)

Example:

For instance, if 180 pounds was your average body weight last week and this week it is 178, then your calculation looks as follows:

(180 − 178) / (180 x 100) = 1.11%

(To calculate, in percentage, how much your body weight changed, you can also use the following application: **http://www.percent-change.com/.** This option is easier if you're having difficulties with the calculation.)

Third, adjust your calorie intake based on your goal and weekly progress. Here's how:

Weight loss: If your body weight doesn't go down or the reduction is below a meaningful rate for more than three consecutive weeks, drop your daily energy intake by 200 calories. A meaningful rate would be an average body weight reduction of 0.5 to 1 percent per week. So, if you're 180 pounds, you should lose between 0.9 and 1.8 pounds per week. If not, reduce your daily energy intake by 200 calories.

Muscle hypertrophy: If your body weight doesn't go up or the increase is below a meaningful rate for more than three consecutive weeks, raise your daily energy intake by 200 calories. A meaningful rate would be an average weight gain between 0.5 to 1 percent for beginner lifters and between 0.4 to 0.8 percent for intermediate and advanced trainees. So, if you're a 180-pound beginner lifter (meaning you have less than one year of proper resistance training experience), you should gain between 0.9 and 1.8 pounds per week. If not, raise your daily energy intake by 200 calories.

How to Track Calorie Intake Effectively and Efficiently

Now that you know how many calories you should consume daily, it's time to start counting calories. Yes, tracking this number is a must because people are terrible at estimating their calorie intake.[28–31] For example, studies show that subjects underestimate how much they eat by as much as 45 percent and underreport their daily energy intake by up to 2,000 calories.[32-33] So, if you don't keep track, you'll likely ruin your progress by consuming more calories than you think you do. Think of that chubby coworker who claims he didn't eat a thing, but for some reason he can't shed those extra pounds.

That's why you count calories. By doing so, you'll know exactly how many calories you consume, and thus you can optimize your number to meet your goals. Moreover, calorie tracking makes you more aware of your food habits and helps you stay on track with your diet.

In fact, prevailing research shows that the mere act of calorie counting can give your results a jump start. As a point of reference, one meta-analysis found that weight-loss programs that use calorie tracking result in, on average, 3.3 kg (7 pounds) more weight loss over a one-year period than plans that don't.[34] And another review study found that those people who track calories are more successful at keeping the lost weight off.[35] The benefits of calorie tracking are also true for gaining weight, by the way. If you monitor your energy intake, you can adjust your food consumption in such a way that you get enough calories each day without overreaching your target. As a result, you'll be more successful at gaining mass and preventing fat gain.

Fortunately, if you have basic working knowledge of a smartphone, calorie counting doesn't have to be a daunting or time-consuming task. There are many apps available that make tracking calories easy. An example is Cronometer (**www.cronometer.com**). Just enter the foods you ate into the free application; it will then calculate how many calories you consumed and show how you're progressing on your daily calorie intake goal.

When it comes to effective calorie tracking, there are three take-home points to keep in mind. First, measure food in its uncooked form because cooking can alter the weight of food. Second, don't rely on measuring cups because volume varies among foods; rather, use a digital scale as this gives more accurate results. Third, keep track of the oils, or whatever you use to cook your food. While many people tend to forget this, it's important because oils are calorie-dense and thus can easily cause you to overreach your energy target.

Borrowing

On certain days, it can be very difficult to maintain your calorie target. Maybe it's because of the grand opening of an artisanal hipster bakery with that bacon-wrapped Mexican coffee doughnut you've heard so much about. Now, you don't want to pass that up, even though you've already hit your daily calorie target. Or perhaps you miscalculated your calorie intake, which led you to exceed your energy target. Or, hey, maybe you had one too many "barley pops" (beers) while working the floor at your favorite single's night. It happens to many of us. Whatever the reason, don't panic—the concept known as borrowing offers a solution.

What is borrowing? It refers to eating slightly more on one day and somewhat less on another, while still hitting your calorie intake goal on a weekly basis. So, let's say that you overate by 300 calories on Monday. In such a case, you can reduce your energy consumption on Tuesday by 300 calories to make up for it. By doing this, you'll still hit your calorie target in the grand scheme of things.

Easy, right? But there are a few crucial things to keep in mind when borrowing. First, avoid raising or lowering your calorie intake by more than 20 percent a day. So, if 2,000 is your daily energy target, don't borrow more than 400 calories on any given day. Second, don't use the concept of borrowing as an excuse to slack on your diet. Rather, use borrowing only when it's impossible or very impractical to stay consistent with your diet that day!

Here is the bottom line: When you start to exceed the 20 percent range, you are no longer borrowing. You are overhauling. Actions have consequences. If you overhaul your daily target calorie count too much or too often, you may be purchasing a ticket to Fat Camp in Soft City (while not a desirable destination, it is a popular one). This strategy of borrowing is for special occasions and unforeseen circumstances, not because you are embarrassed to pop out Tupperware at a lunch meeting or your manager is making Grandma's dumpling recipe.

Key Takeaways

- Calorie balance is the main determining factor for changes to the number on your scale.
- If you want to lose weight (fat), consume fewer calories than you burn. If you want to gain weight (muscle), consume more calories than you burn.
- To determine your ideal daily calorie intake, work through the four-step method outlined above.
- Once you know your daily calorie needs, it's crucial to keep track of your calorie intake because this allows you to hit your daily energy intake target and thus make optimal progress.
- If, due to circumstances, you can't maintain your target calorie target for the day, it's okay to use the borrowing concept—eating slightly more or less on a particular day and compensating on another—as long as you maintain your average calorie goal in the grand scheme of the week.

Step 2: Macros

Here's how to ensure that changes in body weight come in the form of more muscle and less fat, not the other way around.

No one wants to go from big pear to small pear!

Or, to paraphrase boxing great Oscar De La Hoya, there is nothing less attractive than a fat lightweight.

If you go from being large and overweight to being small and chunky, you're still not improving your aesthetic appeal and probably not doing much to help your athletic, or any other kind of, performance.

Unfortunately, if you reduce calories but eat them from low-quality sources, a pear-shaped body will be your "reward." Of course, that's not a true reward, or at least it's not one that anyone would like. Caloric balance is of paramount importance when it comes to changes on the scale. In particular, macronutrient intake is the catalyst for change in your muscle mass or body fat. So, in this section, you'll discover all you need to know about macronutrients, including what they are and how to optimize your intake of them for assistance in reaching your nutritional, fitness, athletic, and even dating goals.

Macronutrients: What Are They and Why Should You Care?

Macronutrients—or macros, for short—are nutrients that provide calories. So, your macro intake determines your calorie consumption. In total, there are four macros. These are protein, carbohydrates, dietary fat, and alcohol. Here's how many calories each of the macros contains:

- Protein: 4 calories per gram
- Carbs: 4 calories per gram
- Dietary fat: 9 calories per gram
- Alcohol: 7 calories per gram

Each macro has a different influence on your body. Let's look closer at each of them.

Protein

Of the macros, protein is most vital for your fitness goals because getting enough of it aids fat loss, supports muscle growth, and helps you recover from workouts.

Protein aids weight loss in a number of ways, with the primary one being that protein is highly filling.[1] It raises various satiety hormones, such as peptide YY, cholecystokinin, and GLP-1, while reducing the "hunger hormone" ghrelin.[1–5] That's why upping protein intake tends to reduce calorie consumption automatically. For example, when subjects in one study raised their protein consumption from 15 to 30 percent of their daily calorie intake, they automatically consumed, on average, 441 fewer calories a day.[6] This led to an average weight loss of 11 pounds in just 12 weeks! Another reason why protein helps you lean down is that it has a high thermogenic effect, meaning that it costs a relatively large number of calories for your body to process and use this macro.

But that's not all. Protein also benefits muscle mass. So if you're on a fat-loss diet, getting enough protein inhibits muscle loss.[7] (You may even gain some if you're a beginner or intermediate lifter, and you diet and exercise right.) And if you're on a mass-gaining plan, getting enough protein helps you with building muscle. In fact, muscle growth is all about building up more proteins—in the form of amino acids—in your muscles than the amount that gets broken down.[8] For this to happen, you must consume enough protein.

How to Set Up Your Protein Intake

Muscle growth: At a minimum, get at least 1.6 grams of protein per kilogram of body weight daily (this translates to 0.73 gram of protein per pound of body weight). This amount optimizes muscle growth, concluded researchers in a 2018 meta-analysis published in the *British Journal of Sports Medicine*.[9] As an anecdotal account, we have seen many use well over one gram of protein per pound of body weight. Yet this is not something that a lot of people in science halls and lab coats discuss, probably because it is difficult to get advanced lifters to participate in research studies. So, if you weigh 80 kilograms (176 pounds), get a minimum of 128 grams of protein daily. Since one gram of protein amounts to four calories, that equals at least 512 calories.

Fat loss: Get between 1.8 and 2.7 grams of protein per kilogram of body weight a day (0.8 and 1.2 grams of protein per pound of body weight).[10] This aids muscle maintenance and reduces hunger cravings while maintaining room for calories from carbs and dietary fat. So, if you weigh 80 kilograms, get between 144 and 216 grams of protein a day. Since one gram of protein amounts to four calories, that's between 576 and 864 calories from protein daily.

Carbs and Dietary Fat

After you've set your protein intake, get the remainder of your calories from carbs and dietary fat. (A small number of calories from alcohol is fine as well, but more on that later.) The reason why we've grouped these two macros together is that there's no optimal intake of them that works best for everyone. Instead, the optimal carb and dietary fat intake varies among individuals.

On the one hand, some people thrive on a high-carb, low-fat approach. On the other hand, as evidenced by the success of our book *Keto Built*, many find their nutritional bliss with a low-carb, high-fat eating style. And for others, a balanced ratio between the two yields optimal results. To find out what's best for you, let's look closer at both macros.

Carbs: The primary benefit of carbs is that they enhance workout performance. Why? When you lift weights, your body mainly uses glucose—the stored form of carbs—for energy.[11] That's why an adequate carb intake aids workout performance.

Dietary fats: This macro is involved in nearly every bodily function, many of which influence your body composition and athletic performance. For example, (the right kind of) dietary fats are essential for insulin functioning and the production of various fat-burning and muscle-building hormones such as human growth hormone and testosterone.[12–15]

How to Set Up Your Intake of Dietary Fat and Carbs

As we've just covered, there's no best carb and dietary fat intake that works for everyone. The optimal ratio between the two depends on various factors, including genetics, activity level, insulin sensitivity, fitness goals, body fat percentage, and others. In a nutshell, here's how you can find out what eating style best fits you—a low-fat/high-carb, high-fat/low-carb, or moderate-carb/moderate-fat diet:

Higher-carb/lower-fat: If you are physically active (e.g., you're an athlete who works out often) or you have a physically demanding job (e.g., you're a construction worker), this approach will fit you well. That's because many physical activities rely primarily on glucose for energy, which is why getting enough carbs aids performance in such situations. Now, this doesn't mean you should remove dietary fats from your diet entirely—that would be a mistake since dietary fats play crucial roles in your health and fitness. Instead, it means that your macro intake will lean more toward the carb end of the spectrum, such as getting 25 percent of your daily calories from protein, 55 percent from carbs, and 20 percent from dietary fat. An example of such a diet is the Parrillo diet.

Lower-carb/higher-fat: Research shows that those who are inactive, have an impaired insulin sensitivity, or exhibit both of these tendencies tend to do best on a high-fat, low-carb approach. This holds true from a health and well-being perspective. Reduced insulin sensitivity can be a result of various factors; examples include being diabetic, having a family history of diabetes, aging, and carrying excess body fat. If you're a woman with polycystic ovarian syndrome (PCOS) or oligomenorrhea (a less frequent menstrual cycle), a high-fat, low-carb approach is also optimal.[15-20] A low-carb diet is typically one that contains fewer than 100 calories a day from carbs. In terms of macros, that generally means consuming about 30 percent of your daily calories from protein, 10 percent from carbs, and 60 percent from dietary fat. Examples of such an eating style are the Paleo diet, Atkins, and the Keto diet.

Contrary to what one might speculate, results don't lie, and many active people and competitive athletes have done very well on Keto, particularly athletes starting with more than 20 percent body fat. While a Keto diet may not be the best call for every athlete, it is something to consider as a possibility.

Moderate-carb/moderate-fat: Those who are moderately active and don't carry excess weight tend to do best on a moderate-carb/moderate-fat eating style. If you fall into this category, simply eat in a balanced fashion by consuming all food groups and hitting your total daily calorie and protein targets. By doing this, you'll automatically consume enough of both macros to reap their benefits. This eating style allows for a lot of flexibility in your diet. An example of a moderate-carb, moderate-fat eating style is the Zone Diet, which is based on a macronutrient intake of 30 percent protein, 40 percent carbs, and 30 percent dietary fat.

Take note that the outlines above are general guidelines. If you truly want to find out your optimal intake of carbs and dietary fat, feel free to experiment with different ratios. For example, try a high-fat, low-carb eating style for three weeks, a low-fat, high-carb approach for three weeks, and a balanced ratio for three weeks. At the end of each three-week period, evaluate how each eating style influenced your hunger levels, body composition, gym performance, sleep quality, and general well-being. By comparing the evaluations, you'll discover which ratio provides you with the best results so that you can continue with that eating style.

Also, consider that the ratio between carbs and dietary fat may differ depending on your goal. If you're on a muscle-building plan, meaning that your calorie intake is elevated, you can get more of both macros. But if you're on a weight-loss diet, your calorie target is reduced, and thus you'll have to cut back on your intake of either carbs, dietary fat, or both. Now, we recommend that you always get at least 50 grams of dietary fat a day because this macro plays such a vital role in health and well-being. Then get the remainder of your calories from whichever eating style fits you best—a high-fat/low-carb, low-fat/high-carb, or moderate-carb/moderate-fat diet.

Alcohol

To look better in that spring break beach pic and to perform your best in athletic pursuits or during modern "courting rituals," it's best to avoid alcohol. Alcohol impairs fat burning, increases fat storage, and raises nitrogen excretion.[21-22] The latter means that it hampers muscle mass; it makes you more prone to muscle loss on a weight-loss diet and impairs growth on a mass-gaining plan.

That said, most people like to have a drink—and then some—once in a while. If that's you, then you may be wondering how to drink alcohol without derailing your fitness progress. Well, good news! There are a few things you can do to minimize the negative effects of alcohol (on your fitness goals, that is; not necessarily on your health, your relationships, and your odd tendency to wake up disrobed on your neighbor's front lawn after "tying one on").

First, limit your relationship with alcohol to moderate consumption up to twice a week at most. Ideally, this would be on a day that you don't work out, to reduce the negative effects alcohol has on recovery and muscle growth. Second, track the macros that are in your beverages, and count alcoholic calories toward your carb intake. Third, try to limit alcohol consumption to at most two drinks. However, even though it's not ideal, it's okay to go over this amount once in a while, if you still hit your macros and don't make it a habit.

The bottom line is power drinking impairs power building.

How to Track Macronutrients

When it comes to tracking macros, there are many apps available that make this process faster and more convenient. As outlined in the previous chapter, Cronometer (**www.cronometer.com**) is an example of such an app. Simply log your food consumption into the application, and it will automatically calculate your macro intake.

Key Takeaways

- Macros have a significant influence on whether lost or gained weight comes as muscle mass or body fat.
- Protein is the most essential macro. To build muscle, consume a minimum of 0.73 gram of protein per pound of body weight a day. To lose fat, consume between 0.8 and 1.2 grams of protein per pound of body weight.
- The optimal intake of carb and dietary fat varies among individuals, with activity levels being the primary influencer.
- While alcohol is best avoided, if you want to drink, limit your alcohol consumption to at most two glasses twice a week, and count alcoholic calories toward your carb intake.
- Measure your daily macro intake with a tracking app such as Cronometer (**www.chronometer.com**) or MyFitnessPal (**www.myfitnesspal.com**).

Step 3: Food Selection

Learn the truth about which foods you should consume to boost diet adherence, slash hunger cravings, and skyrocket your results.

While calories and macros form the foundation of every successful body transformation diet, food selection follows closely in importance. In this section, you'll discover the three main reasons why you should pay attention to food selection, and you'll learn which foods you should consume for optimal results, based on your situation and goals.

Hint: When it comes to the calories and macros you consume, processed food from the local quickie mart ain't going to cut the mustard.

The Three Main Reasons Why It's Vital to Consume the Right Foods

First, certain foods are more filling than others. And if you mostly consume satiating foods, you'll suffer fewer cravings, and thus it'll be easier to keep your calorie intake under control.

One interesting study that shows how food selection influences hunger and calorie intake was published in the *American Journal of Clinical Nutrition* way back in 1983.[1] In the study, 20 subjects could eat as much as they desired for five days on two different diets (a diet made up of foods high in energy density and a diet of foods low in energy density). The high-energy diet contained calorie-dense foods such as desserts and meats. The low-energy diet was made up of low-calorie foods, such as vegetables, fruits, dried beans, and grains.

The result? While the subjects could eat to their heart's content on both diets, food intake and hunger levels varied significantly between the eating styles. On the low-energy diet, the participants felt full after consuming an average of 1,570 calories. But to achieve the same satiety on the high-energy diet, they had to consume 3,000 calories. That's almost double the number of calories!

What's more, another study compared the satiety effects of 38 foods, which led to some interesting findings. For example, even though croissants contain five times more calories than boiled potatoes, the latter was found to be seven times more satiating. [2] In other words, it'll be much easier to obtain and maintain a healthy weight if you get your calories from boiled potatoes than from croissants.

To give you an example, below are two diets containing roughly 2,300 calories. Diet One is made up of calorie-dense foods and thus would not be ideal for weight loss. The second diet contains low-energy but highly satiating foods and is an example of a proper fat-loss diet.

Diet One:

Meal	Food + Serving	Calories
#1	McDonald's Big Mac (one serving)	541
	Coca-Cola (one large bottle)	273
#2	French fries (300 grams)	471
	Mayonnaise (2 tbsp)	280
#3	Chicken nuggets (150 grams)	465
	Vanilla ice cream (100 grams)	310
Total Number of Calories: 2,340		

Diet Two:

Meal	Food + Serving	Calories
#1	Eggs, whole, hard-boiled (3 medium)	205
	Apple, fresh, with skin (1 medium)	95
	Greek yogurt, plain, nonfat with fresh blueberries (300 grams + 75 grams)	220
	Coffee, prepared from grounds	5
#2	Caesar salad with shrimp (300 grams)	313
	Avocado, Hass (1 medium)	227
	Strawberries, raw (250 grams)	80
#3	Salmon (200 grams)	364
	Green beans (200 grams)	70
	Boiled potatoes (200 grams)	152
	Lemon (1 medium)	17
	Crème fraîche, reduced-fat (200 grams)	326
#4	Whey protein shake (1 scoop of 31 grams)	124
	Banana (1 medium)	105
Total number of calories: 2,303		

Second, the amount of vitamins, minerals, trace minerals, and other beneficial compounds varies among foods. This matters because most of these compounds influence bodily functions related to your figure and athletic performance, such as hormone and energy production and fat oxidation.

Zinc is an example of such a nutrient. Getting enough of this mineral is vital for many bodily functions related to your figure, including the production of testosterone, a hormone that has a vast influence on muscle growth and fat burning. Time and again, research shows that a zinc deficiency can significantly reduce testosterone levels in men.[3] In other words, not getting enough zinc can make you physically flaccid and reduce fat burning, muscle growth, and athletic performance by impairing testosterone levels.

What's more, zinc is also essential for your metabolic rate. Not getting enough of the mineral can downregulate metabolism. This means that you'll burn fewer calories each day, making it harder to obtain and maintain ideal body weight. Hence, a case study published in *Annals of Nutrition and Metabolism* found that a zinc-deficient female was able to raise her resting metabolic rate by 527 calories a day just by supplementing with the mineral for two months.[4] That equals 3,689 calories a week, which, energy-wise, represents more than what's found in one pound of pure body fat.[5]

Zinc is just one example of the many vitamins, minerals, and trace minerals that influence your figure. Other examples include iron, which is crucial for energy production and workout performance; calcium, which supports metabolism and fat oxidation; and potassium, which helps eliminate water retention.

Third, certain foods are more beneficial for health than others. Now, if you mainly eat these healthy foods, you'll feel more vigorous and vital. As a result, you'll have more energy and motivation to go to the gym, stick to your diet, and still be up for an active "personal life."

Moreover, maintaining a healthy diet will reduce your chance of getting sick. This is important because if you're sick, you can't work out (at least not optimally). Missing your workouts or training at a lower level may reduce your progress and cause you to lose your gains, especially if you're sick over a long time frame.

Don't lose your gains.

How to Optimize Food Selection

When you're shopping for food at the market, one applicable approach to food selection is to stay on the perimeter (in other words, avoid aisles filled with the processed, sugar-heavy options). This will allow you to select foods that are filled with your daily nutrients and support your fitness goals. Remember to get at least 80 percent of your foods from whole, nutritious sources such as fruits, vegetables, meat, fish, nuts, seeds, and healthy oils. Consume a bare minimum of four servings of fruits and vegetables a day and shoot for more than five. In addition, maintain a varied diet so that you get a wide range of nutrients.

Focusing on nutrient-dense, low-calorie foods is especially important on a fat-loss diet because it aids hunger control, making it easier to maintain your calorie target. When your goal is dropping body fat, get your protein intake by consuming primarily lean protein sources like chicken and tuna. This helps to keep your calorie intake in control. In addition, avoid starchy carbs such as white rice and bread because they provide many calories without satiating hunger effectively.

When you're on a muscle-building diet, you should still consume primarily nutrient-dense foods. However, since gaining weight requires an increased calorie intake, it's okay to consume more energy-dense foods (as long as you don't overreach your calorie target). Remember, even if you're looking to gain weight, if the cashier at your local chain fast-food spot knows you by name, this is an indication that you should dial back on the junk food.

Examples of energy-dense foods are starchy carbs (rice, quinoa, oatmeal, etc.), fattier cuts of meat (beef, pork, lamb), higher-fat dairy (full-fat milk, full-fat yogurt, cheese, etc.), and nuts and seeds. Adding those foods into your diet is especially helpful if you have difficulty consuming enough calories.

To make sure that you get enough of each vitamin and mineral, it is best to get a blood panel test done to evaluate your levels of each micronutrient. But since that may be pricey and inconvenient, an alternative is tracking your food intake with the app Cronometer (**www.cronometer.com**). If you log your food into the app, it automatically calculates your intake of essential vitamins and minerals. Now, if it turns out that you regularly consume too little of a specific micronutrient, then adjust your intake accordingly. Just search online for foods that are rich in that particular nutrient and add one or more of them into your diet. For example, if your zinc intake is subpar, then consuming oysters, lamb, or pumpkin seeds can offer the solution. Also, taking the nutrient in supplement form or consuming a high-quality multivitamin is beneficial for reaching your daily nutritional needs.

Key Takeaways

- Food selection is crucial for three main reasons: Certain foods are more filling than others; nutrition content varies among foods; and each food affects health differently.
- To ensure that you get enough of each vitamin and mineral, track your food intake with Cronometer (***www.cronometer.com***).
- If necessary, adjust your food intake to reach your daily nutrient needs, supplement with a particular vitamin or mineral of which you're not getting enough, or take a multivitamin.

Step 4: Meal Frequency

Discover the exact meal frequency you should follow to boost diet adherence and supercharge your results.

Meal frequency is controversial.

Old-school bodybuilders claim you have to eat six meals per day, while the New Age intermittent-fasting guru (with the man bun and esoteric body art) is all about that daily-single-meal life.

So, with all these conflicting opinions, what is the best meal frequency to reach your goals? And at what times should you get in those feedings? In this section, you'll discover the unbiased, evidence-based approach backed by science. But, more importantly, this is material that has been proven "in the trenches" of training halls and hard-core gyms. Then, most importantly, we'll look at the best feeding schedule for your situation and goals.

Most Things You've Been Told about Meal Frequency Are Wrong

Your muscle-building salvation or fat-loss damnation does not depend on meal frequency. This topic is not irrelevant, but it is far from being the central focus of your nutritional plan.

This is true whether you want to lose or gain weight. For example, researchers found that meal frequency doesn't influence body weight when calorie intake is matched.[1–2] So, as long as you eat the same number of calories, your weight is not influenced by the number of meals over which you spread this food. The same is also true for metabolism. Contrary to popular belief, it makes no difference to your metabolic rate whether you wolf down all your daily calories in one sitting or nibble them throughout the day.[3] As long as your food intake is identical, your metabolism remains the same.

In regard to being consistent with your food consumption, remember a central decree from the original *Jailhouse Strong* book: The body thrives on a routine.

But that's not all. When it comes to muscle growth, the old-school bodybuilding wisdom on the topic of meal frequency is that you have to eat every three hours. Now there are not a lot of studies supporting this claim. But it is important to recognize that success leaves a trail, and this method has been implemented by many successful athletes. While it could be the routine of eating at the same time daily that leads to positive results, we should recognize that success (whether it's documented by scientific findings or not) often offers strategies worthy of emulation.

According to many studies, unless you consume fewer than two meals a day, how often you eat does not influence muscle mass.[4] So, to be safe, as long as you consume at least three meals a day (like Arnold's mentor, Reg Park) and spread out your protein intake evenly over these feedings, you'll be okay.[5]

How to Set Up Your Feeding Frequency for Optimal Progress

While meal frequency doesn't influence your results directly (unless you consume a very low meal frequency, that is), it can affect your results indirectly. The primary reason for this is that meal frequency impacts appetite and diet adherence. In other words, with certain meal frequencies, you'll suffer fewer hunger cravings, and thus it'll be easier to stay on track with your diet (we believe this is one of the reasons why the bodybuilding approach is so successful). So, here's what we recommend to you:

Weight loss: If you want to lean down, consume between three and five meals a day. This frequency offers an excellent balance between relatively satiating meals and regular ones. You want to avoid going above this range on a weight-loss diet because doing so tends to reduce the size of each meal to such an extent that each feeding becomes very small and unsatiating, which, in turn, increases the risk of overeating. Consuming fewer than a minimum of three meals can be an issue because you have to go for extended periods without food. This can encourage bingeing. In addition, while going below three meals a day will not necessarily change your weight, it may increase muscle wasting. So, in short, spread out your food intake over three, four, or five meals a day.

Muscle growth: If you want to gain mass, our general recommendation is also to consume between three and five meals a day. However, if you want to build muscle and have difficulty consuming enough calories, then it's fine to raise your meal frequency to six, seven, or eight feedings a day because eating more often makes it easier to consume more calories.

Consistency

Remember, the body thrives on a routine. For optimal health and fitness, remain consistent with your eating pattern, as irregular meal patterns worsen blood lipid profile levels and insulin sensitivity.[6-7] So, for example, don't consume three meals on day one, five the day after, and then fall back to four feedings. Instead, choose a specific meal frequency and try to stick to it as best you can. For the best results, make a plan that you'll stick with—for instance, you might decide to consume four meals a day, one at 9 am, noon, 5 pm, and 9 pm—and stay with it.

Key Takeaways

- Unless you consume fewer than two meals a day, meal frequency doesn't directly influence body composition; however, it does *indirectly* affect body composition, primarily by impacting hunger levels.
- On a fat-loss plan, consume between three and five meals per day. On a muscle-building plan, eat between three and eight meals a day.
- Avoid irregular eating patterns. Instead, choose a specific meal frequency and stick to it as best you can.

Step 5: Nutrient Timing

Discover the evidence-based truth about nutrient timing to maximize your workout performance and sex appeal.

Should you consume a protein shake immediately after your workout?

Is the post-workout drink pitched by the perky blonde at the mall going to get you more jacked?

Are carbs best avoided before bedtime if you want to get shredded? Or are such bits of advice on nutrient timing just baloney?

In this section, you'll discover the evidence-based answers to such questions. We're going to tackle whether nutrient timing is important and, if so, how you can optimize it.

Is Nutrient Timing Important?

Nutrient timing refers to the time at which you consume your foods. And while this dieting factor receives much attention in the fitness world, the truth is that when you consume specific nutrients isn't that important.[1] Here's what a review study published in the *Journal of the International Society of Sports Nutrition* concluded: "...alterations in nutrient timing and frequency appear to have little effect on fat loss or lean mass retention." In other words, never let nutrient timing distract you from the more vital nutrition fundamentals such as calorie and macro intake and food quality.

That said, once you have the dieting fundamentals, such as calorie intake and food selection, in check, optimizing nutrition timing may give you a slight edge. In fact, the leaner and more muscular you currently are, the more important nutrient timing becomes. This is because the closer you get to your genetic ceiling, the more influential smaller factors become to continue progress. So, after controlling the previous steps, here's how to approach nutrient timing:

How to Time Your Nutrients for Optimal Results

Pre-workout: If you consumed a protein-rich meal a few hours before your workout, you don't need to consume pre-workout protein within an hour or so before your workout; it has no, or at best only a tiny, benefit on muscle growth.[2] The reason for this is that you still have amino acids from the meal you ate a few hours earlier in your bloodstream. After all, it takes several hours—around two to six hours for most feedings—before your body fully absorbs the nutrients of a meal.[3]

That said, in some scenarios it's beneficial to do an extra protein feeding around an hour before your session. One such situation is when you follow an intermittent-fasting eating style. In such a case it's beneficial because you didn't consume protein a few hours beforehand. Another reason to consume pre-workout protein is to be on the safe side. Since it won't hinder your gains and at best may help slightly, there's nothing wrong with consuming some protein an hour before kicking off your workout. Regarding the dosage, 25 to 30 grams between 30 and 60 minutes before your session will help you to reap all the (potential) benefits.

When it comes to pre-workout dietary fats and carbs, the first macro doesn't provide benefits when consumed pre-workout.[4] So you don't have to consume dietary fat before your exercise session. Pre-workout carbs, however, can be beneficial because they aid workout performance by supplying your body with an extra energy source.[5-6] Be aware that not everyone sees a boost in performance in response to consuming pre-workout carbs. In particular, those who thrive on a ketogenic diet might even feel sluggish with pre-workout carbs. Nonetheless, there are many who benefit from this, so you may want to test it. The idea is to consume somewhere around 20 or more grams of carbs before your workout session. You can get those carbs from either food or a sports drink.

Intra-workout: This refers to consuming nutrients during your workout. Generally speaking, intra-workout nutrition is not essential, if you get enough protein in general and some before your workout. That said, if you feel light-headed during your workout, consuming a fast-acting carb source such as a sports drink often helps. Otherwise, don't worry about intra-workout nutrition.

Post-workout: If you consumed protein before your session, you don't need to consume post-workout nutrients as soon as possible. It takes a few hours before the nutrients from a meal reach your bloodstream, so you'll have enough amino acids floating through your veins, ready to be taken up by the cells in your muscles. The same holds true for consuming carbs immediately after your session—it's not necessary for optimal recovery and growth (although there's nothing wrong with it either if your macros allow it).[7] An exception is if you worked out strenuously for more than an hour. In such a case, a fast-acting protein source such as whey can be beneficial.

Pre-bed: Consuming protein before going to sleep can be beneficial because it aids muscle growth.[8-9] Besides, you may also want to consume some of your daily carb intake a few hours before hitting the sack. Doing so raises serotonin levels in your brain, which helps you fall asleep more quickly.[10] As a side note, this is why we recommend cheat meals or refeeds at night on a ketogenic diet. Also, some dietary fat is okay as it helps with stabilizing blood sugar levels, which makes you less likely to wake up in the middle of the night. In other words, consume a protein-rich, balanced meal a few hours before going to bed.

Carb Cycling

Carb cycling is a popular eating style among lifters. It is based on consuming more carbs but less dietary fat on workout days, and doing the opposite on days you rest (fewer carbs, more dietary fat). A favorite among bodybuilding and fat-loss coaches, the idea behind carb cycling is that it expedites fat loss and muscle growth due to its effect on insulin. In a nutshell, the increased carb intake on workout days raises insulin levels, which is thought to aid muscle growth.[11] On the other hand, the reduced carb intake on rest days lowers insulin, which should enhance fat burning since insulin impairs fat burning (antilipolytic).

Although there's no hard research on this eating style, it would be irresponsible to completely dismiss it. The bottom line is that following carb cycling won't impede your results, and it potentially will give you a slight boost in performance. It could even help you look better naked.

While there are different approaches to carb cycling, here's what we recommend you do: Split up your weekly macro intake between high-carb and low-carb days. Then, on workout days, consume most of your calories (protein excluded) from carbs and limit your intake of dietary fat to at most 60 grams. And on rest days, limit your carb intake to at most 100 grams and get the majority of your calories from dietary fat.

Intermittent Fasting

Intermittent fasting is based on an eating pattern in which you abstain from eating for the greater part of the day and consume all your foods in a smaller "feeding window." A popular approach is fasting for 16 hours a day and consuming all calories in an 8-hour time frame. Now, while intermittent fasting has gained much popularity, it doesn't have any huge benefits for fat loss or muscle growth. That said, following such an eating style can still be beneficial because many people find it easier to control their calorie intake if they shorten their feeding window. For example, studies show that skipping breakfast (which is a form of intermittent fasting) can reduce daily energy intake by up to 400 calories.[12–14] And another study found that when non-breakfast eaters were instructed to consume breakfast, they consumed, on average, 266 more calories a day over a four-week period. This caused an average weight gain of 0.7 kilogram.[15]

Because intermittent fasting tends to reduce calorie consumption and make it easier to keep food intake in control, it can be particularly beneficial for those who are on a weight-loss plan. So if you want to lean down, feel free to experiment with such an eating style. A pattern that we recommend is a 16-hour fasting window for men and a 14-hour fasting window for women daily. In the remaining hours—an 8-hour window for males and a 10-hour window for females—consume all of your food. (The rest of your diet, such as your calorie and macro intake, remains; you just change the timing at which you eat your foods.) The reason why a longer feeding window is recommended for females is that some women respond less favorably to more extended periods of fasting. Intermittent fasting is safe for healthy individuals and linked to various health benefits. However, if, as a woman, you notice that this eating style negatively affects your menstrual cycle (as some women do), stop your intermittent fasting and go back to a "regular" feeding style immediately.

If your goal is to build muscle and gain weight, intermittent fasting tends to be less beneficial. This is not because such an eating style impairs muscle growth, as some claim. It does not. Rather, it is because intermittent fasting can make it tougher to reach your daily calorie surplus. After all, intermittent fasting tends to reduce calorie intake automatically. Now, if you have a big appetite and no problems with reaching your calorie goal, this won't be a problem. But if you find it hard to get in enough calories, avoid an intermittent-fasting eating style as it makes reaching your daily energy target only harder.

On the road to getting jacked and packing on pounds, intermittent fasting would be the scenic route. We suggest a more direct option.

Key Takeaways

- While nutrient timing is not essential, optimizing this factor may slightly enhance your results, especially if you're an advanced athlete.
- Intra-workout nutrition is usually unnecessary.
- If you consume enough protein in general and had some within a few hours before your workout, protein immediately post-workout is superfluous (unless you train hard for an extended

time; then it's beneficial). Consuming carbs or dietary fats immediately post-workout isn't necessary either.
- Consume a balanced meal a few hours before going to bed to aid muscle growth and recovery and sleep quality.
- Although research is lacking, carb cycling may assist muscle growth and fat loss.
- Intermittent fasting can help with controlling calorie intake, making it beneficial for losing weight.

Step 6: Hydration

Nail this down to enhance your figure, upgrade your workout performance, and make dieting significantly easier.

Hydration is rarely talked about in the fitness world. That's a shame because being hydrated is crucial for your physique and training performance. In this section, we'll cover why that's the case, and you'll also discover how much water you should drink to conquer your fitness goals.

So grab some water, start reading, and get ready to look broader and better for the family beach vacation or the date that ends the right way.

The Importance of Hydration

Your body is made up of around 60 to 70 percent water. This water is present in all your cells, organs, and tissues to support proper functioning and temperature regulation. In other words, water is crucial for surviving, let alone thriving. The problem? Most of us are chronically dehydrated. While it's hard to put a figure on dehydration prevalence, a survey of 3,003 Americans found that 75 percent likely had a net fluid loss, leading to chronic dehydration.[1] Such a lack of bodily fluid levels can have severe side effects, not only on your health but also on your athletic performance and how you look in the buff.

Astonishingly, those who don't drink water habitually consume, on average, 9 percent more calories daily than those who do.[2] For an average adult male (based on an energy need of 2,500 calories), that represents around 1,575 more calories a week, which, energy-wise, equals roughly 0.45 pound of pure fat.[3] The reason why dehydration increases calorie intake—and thereby raises the risk of weight and fat gain—is that your brain can't effectively distinguish the difference between thirst and hunger. So being dehydrated may cause you to reach for a meal even though what you need is a glass of water.

But that's not all! Dehydration also hampers athletic performance. Mild dehydration of just 3 to 4 percent of body mass loss reduces strength by around 2 percent (that's roughly 12 pounds off a 600-pound deadlift), and more severe dehydration lowers performance even further.[4–5] Dehydration impairs performance because it reduces motivation, raises fatigue, alters body temperature control, and makes exercise feel a lot harder, both physically and mentally.[6] The result? Because you won't be able to train optimally in the gym, you can't maximally stimulate your muscles, which leads to diminished progress.

Staying hydrated is also crucial for muscle growth. One reason for this is that muscles are made up of about 75 to 80 percent water. That's why a hydrated muscle looks fuller and larger compared to a dehydrated one. Plus, research also shows that muscle cell hydration status influences protein synthesis and breakdown rates.[7] In other words, getting enough water aids muscle growth.

How to Calculate Your Daily Water Intake Needs

There's no set-in-stone number on optimal water intake, because we all have different fluid intake needs due to various factors such as body size, activity levels, and the environment we're in. That's why it's not ideal to aim to consume a specified amount of water each day. Instead, to figure out how much water you should drink for optimal health and fitness progress, it's better to evaluate your urination habits. This allows you to see if you're getting enough water. How do you do this? It's simple. Aim for at least five clear urinations a day. That is five urinations during which your urine is clear; not five in total! You want your urine to be clear and copious, at least five times daily. If you accomplish that, you're well-hydrated. If not, you need to consume more water.

If you're not getting enough water daily, one excellent way to raise your intake of it is to consume one glass of water before each meal. So if you eat four meals per day, for example, that would raise your daily water intake by around 800 milliliters. But besides raising your water intake, drinking a glass of water before your meal also has another benefit: It can increase feelings of fullness and thereby reduce your total calorie intake. This is because water consumption causes your stomach wall to stretch, which signals to your brain that your stomach is fuller. For example, one study on obese older adults found that drinking 500 milliliters of water 30 minutes before breakfast decreased calorie consumption by an average of 13 percent.[8]

Key Takeaways

- Inadequate water intake hampers body shape in various ways. These include raising hunger and calorie intake, reducing workout performance, and impairing muscle growth.
- Many people fail to consume enough water, causing them to be in a chronic state of dehydration.
- While there's no optimal water intake for everyone due to individual and environmental differences, an excellent guideline to ensure proper hydration is making sure you have at least five clear urinations a day.
- If you're having difficulty consuming enough water, start by drinking a glass of it before every meal.

Step 7: Diet Breaks and Refeeds

Here's how to alleviate the downsides of dieting and boost your fat-loss efforts by strategically overeating.

Refeeds and diet breaks are powerful tools to boost fat loss and make dieting less tedious. Unfortunately, most dieters use them incorrectly or not at all. In this section, you'll discover what refeeds and diet breaks are, why you want to use them, and how to do so the right way.

So, you'll learn how, why, and when to hit your favorite all-you-can-eat buffet.

Note: Refeeds and diet breaks are relevant only if you're on a weight-loss diet. If you're on a mass-gaining plan, refeeds are not recommended. We'll explain below.

The Problem with Dieting

Your body is a dynamic organism continually adapting to your food intake. This is especially true when you're on a fat-loss plan. To be clear, if you take in fewer calories than you burn, your body will adjust certain functions to slow down your weight loss or even stop it. These include raising your hunger level while slowing your metabolism. One study found that subjects who had just lost 10 percent of their body weight had, on average, an 18 percent lower metabolic rate than those of the same body weight who hadn't recently dieted.[1] The reason your body adjusts while you're in a calorie-deficit state is most likely linked back to hunter-gatherer times. In that environment, you never know when the next meal will be available, so your body wants to hold onto mass because it acts as an energy reserve for when food is scarce.

While these adaptations were beneficial for our ancestors to ensure survival, they aren't very relevant (for most of us) in the modern world. For the majority of our readers, your next meal is almost always within reach. If it's not immediately available, a simple call is all it takes to get junk food delivered to your door. Be grateful, thankful, and appreciative for the surplus of calories readily available to you.

Moving forward with gratitude, it is important to recognize that these modern adaptations may cause more problems than they fix. In fact, the easy access to calories is one of the main reasons why, despite good intentions, nearly all dieters fail to lose weight and keep it off. After all, the dieting-induced metabolic slowdown means that you must further reduce your calorie intake to keep on losing weight. And while eating less is hard in general, it's even tougher when you are on a weight-loss plan where your hunger levels are already elevated and food seems to be all around you.

Note: Your body also adapts to a calorie surplus, although to a significantly lesser extent. In fact, the metabolism of some people doesn't raise at all in response to overeating.[2] The reason why your body adjusts less—or not at all—is probably because gaining some (a slight increase in pounds, rather than a gut hanging over your waistline) extra weight would be beneficial during hunter-gatherer times, because it acts as an energy reserve for when food is scarce.

The Solution?

While dieting-induced adaptations can make weight loss more challenging, fortunately, there's something you can do to reduce or even eliminate the adverse effects: strategic overfeeding. In other words, revving up your calorie intake for a certain amount of time. This benefits your weight-loss results in various ways, such as raising metabolism, refilling muscle glycogen stores for enhanced workout performance, aiding hormonal health, reducing dieting-induced water retention, and reducing appetite and cravings.[3-7] Moreover, raising your food intake once in a while also gives you a break from dieting, making it easier to stay on track with your fat-loss plan. Now, when it comes to overfeeding strategically, there are two methods that can be helpful to aid your fat-loss efforts. These are diet breaks and refeeds. Let's break down each of them.

Diet Breaks

This is a one- or two-week time frame during which you go off your weight-loss eating plan and eat at a calorie-maintenance level instead (again, this refers to the level of caloric consumption where you're neither losing nor gaining weight). This "resets" your metabolism, undoes other dieting-induced adaptations, and gives your mind a rest from being on a diet. For these reasons, diet breaks may even help you lose fat, as found by a recent study published in the *International Journal of Obesity*.[8] For the study, 51 obese men were randomly split up into two groups. One group followed an ongoing calorie-restricted diet for 16 weeks in total. The other group alternated between the same calorie-restricted diet and two-week diet breaks, during which they ate at calorie maintenance. This latter group followed this cycle for 30 weeks in total (16 weeks of restricting calorie intake and 14 weeks of maintaining the diet break protocol), meaning that both groups maintained the calorie-restricted diet for the same length, which was 16 weeks. The result? Those who did diet breaks lost, on average, 11 pounds more, and they were also more successful at keeping the lost weight off.

How to use a diet break: Even though the group who did diet breaks in the study mentioned above lost more weight, they also needed nearly double the amount of time to complete 16 weeks of calorie-restricted dieting. So, you want to use diet breaks in such a way that they give you the best return on your investment. A good model is after following a calorie-restricted diet for 8 to 10 weeks, take a 2-week break for maintenance-level calorie consumption. Then go back to reducing calories.

Doing a diet break is simple. Just calculate your calorie-maintenance intake and eat according to this amount for two weeks. You can figure this number out by going back to chapter one and going through the calculations. (Skip steps three and four of the formula because those aren't relevant in this case.) Then, consume around one gram of protein per pound of body weight and get the rest of your calories from carbs and dietary fat in a ratio that fits your preferences. (A small number of calories from alcohol is okay as well, but limit this amount according to the guidelines in the section on macros.) After you finish your diet break, continue your regular calorie-restricted diet to kick-start fat loss again.

Important notes: Everyone responds differently to diet breaks. While some people lose weight during a diet break (that's mainly water loss), others have the number on the scale go up during such a phase. Now, if you eat at calorie maintenance, such a possible rise in weight is not due to fat gain. Instead, it's because of an increase in muscle glycogen storage and intramuscular water retention. Once you start to reduce your calorie intake again, you'll lose this weight. So don't worry about this sudden spike. Also, the concept of refeeding—which we'll discuss in the next section—doesn't apply during a diet break, so don't do one of those.

Refeeds

Like a diet break, a refeed is a time frame during which you rev up your calorie intake. The main difference, however, is that a refeed lasts a shorter time (typically between 1 and 48 hours). Due to this reduced window, refeeds cause a less severe "reset" of your metabolism, hormonal status, and hunger levels (although it is still to a very beneficial extent). However, they also require less time, which means that you can get back on track with your fat-loss plan faster.

How to use refeeds: If you are on a fat-loss plan, use refeeds to boost your results. How often you do a refeed depends on your body fat percentage. If you are a man above 15 percent body fat or a woman above 23 percent body fat, refeed once every 14 days. If you are a man with a body fat percentage below 15 percent or a woman below 23 percent body fat, refeed once every seven days. You want to refeed more often as you get leaner because you are more prone to dieting-induced adaptations. It is important that you plan in advance the day and time you will do this refeed.

On your refeed day, raise your calorie intake by 30 percent above your regular consumption. So, if you are dieting on 2,100 calories a day, consume 2,730 calories during your refeed. Whether you spread those extra calories out over the day or take them all at one sitting is up to you. Both are fine, although most people note that consuming all the extra calories in one meal is most satiating. That is, one trip to your favorite local all-you-can-eat can be cathartic on both a nutritional and emotional level.

When it comes to your macro intake during your refeed, here is what to do: First, consume between 0.8 and 1.2 grams of protein per pound of body weight. (That's the same number that you should consume anyway, as outlined in the macronutrient chapter.) Second, keep your dietary fat intake below 60 grams. Do this because dietary fat isn't effective at raising leptin—one of the main goals of doing a refeed—and because this macro is most likely to be stored as body fat during a refeed.[9] Third, minimize alcohol consumption as this macro inhibits leptin.[10] If you want to consume a beverage, go for one standard-size drink at most and count the calories toward your total energy intake. Fourth, get the remainder of your calories from carbs. You want to do this for the following three reasons: This macro most significantly raises leptin levels; it refills muscle glycogen stores (which naturally decline on a weight-loss plan) and thereby aids workout performance; and this macro is least likely to be stored as body fat during a refeed.[11-12]

Key Takeaways

- If you're on a weight-loss plan, your body will adapt to prevent you from losing too much weight too fast. It does this by downregulating metabolism, raising hunger levels, and reducing motivation to work out and move.
- These bodily changes make it harder and harder to lose weight once you get leaner.

- Doing diet breaks and refeeds will reduce the severity of these adaptations.
- On a weight-loss plan, do a diet break once every 8 to 10 weeks of calorie-restricted dieting according to the guidelines above.
- On a weight-loss plan, do a refeed once every 14 days if you're are a man above 15 percent body fat or a woman above 23 percent, and once every 7 days if you are a man with a body fat percentage below 15 percent or a woman below 23 percent body fat, according to the guideline above.

Step 8: Supplements

Upgrade your results with the right supplements—without wasting money on useless or harmful pills and powders.

Regardless of what the kid working the counter at your local supplement store will tell you, no pill, powder, or potion will undo a bad nutrition plan and magically turn your body into that of a fitness magazine cover model.

Supplements cannot make a pit bull out of a poodle.

In reality, supplements are a luxury, not a necessity, for losing fat, building muscle, and optimizing your athletic performance. Instead, the key to reaching such goals will always be maintaining a proper diet, working out hard and smart, and getting enough quality rest and recovery. But limited value is still some value, and the more advanced you are, the more certain supplements can give you a small advantage in reaching the goals you've set for your physique and athletic performance. In this section, you'll discover seven supplements that are proven to be beneficial in specific scenarios.

The Seven Supplements That Can Support Your Success

Whey protein: As we've already covered, getting enough protein is crucial for reaching your fitness goals. This is true whether you want to lose fat, build muscle, or enhance athletic performance. But what if you can't get enough protein through diet alone? That's when whey protein powder can offer the solution.

Whey is a by-product from cheese manufacturing. It's the liquid that is left after milk has been strained and curdled. This high-protein liquid then gets spray-dried into a powder and undergoes microfiltration. What you are left with is whey protein powder.

The main advantage of whey over a food source is that nearly all the calories come from protein. So whey can help you reach your protein goal without providing many extra calories. The reason why we recommend whey among all the available protein powder variations is that it has, along with casein, the best amino acid profile for muscle growth and the highest bioavailability.[1] Besides, whey is also one of the cheapest options. However, even though whey is our top pick, if, for whatever reason, you want to use another protein powder form, then we recommend either casein, egg white, or pea protein powder. (The latter is plant-based, so if you follow a vegan diet or don't respond well to dairy products, pea protein powder will be a good alternative.)

Creatine: Creatine is a molecule that is naturally found in your muscles. Your body can produce creatine out of the amino acids arginine, glycine, and methionine, and you can also get some through food. Now, the reason why creatine is an exciting supplement is that much research shows supplementing with this molecule is a safe and effective way to boost muscle growth and strength gains. For example, one review involving 22 studies found that creatine monohydrate supplementation increased the number of repetitions subjects could do during resistance training with a sub-maximal load by 14 percent.[2] And another meta-analysis found that, in combination with resistance training, creatine had the most profound impact on muscle growth among 250 evaluated supplements (six supplements had more than two studies that fulfilled the criteria for inclusion in the meta-analysis).[3]

There are various reasons why creatine helps strength gains and muscle growth. Those include—but are not limited to—supporting energy production, increasing muscle cellular hydration, and aiding the production of various muscle-building hormones, including testosterone.[4]

If you want to supplement with creatine, take 3 to 5 grams of creatine monohydrate daily. You can also do a loading phase during which you supplement daily with 20 to 25 grams for five days before going back to the regular dosage. This will saturate your muscle creatine stores faster, and thus you'll see a sharper rise in strength, power, and body weight. However, such a phase is not necessary, because you'll achieve the same results by taking a smaller dosage over a prolonged period. Also, please note that you may gain a few pounds of weight throughout the first few weeks of supplementation. Unless you go overboard with your diet, this is not body fat. Instead, it's an increase in water weight inside your muscle cells.

Caffeine: This stimulatory and anti-sleep compound, which is most often extracted from coffee beans, is a cheap and effective way to aid athletic performance. (Not to mention that a morning cup is linked to many health benefits.) Supplementing with caffeine can support workout performance by suppressing fatigue and improving power output, aerobic and anaerobic exercise capacity, and focus.[5-9] Besides, caffeine can also aid fat loss by enhancing metabolism, although this effect is small.

Now, it's important to note that caffeine delivers performance-enhancing and fat-loss benefits only if you're not tolerant to the compounds. So, if you want to use caffeine to aid performance and fat loss, you should limit caffeine use to only once or twice per week. If you've already built up a tolerance to caffeine, abstaining from it for two weeks will resensitize your body to the benefits.

To use caffeine as a fat burner, take 200 milligrams of caffeine, ideally before a workout. To use caffeine as a performance enhancer, take between 4 to 6 milligrams per kilogram of body weight 30 minutes before your workout. So, if you weigh 68 kilograms (150 pounds), supplement with 272 to 408 milligrams of caffeine. You can get this caffeine either in a supplement (pill or powder form) or through a caffeinated beverage such as coffee. Because caffeine can interrupt sleep, it's best to consume it before 2 p.m. (or at least nine hours before going to bed, if you have an altered sleeping schedule).

Citrulline: Citrulline is an amino acid that was first found in watermelon. It can aid athletic performance, which it primarily does by raising nitric oxide levels.[10] Nitric oxide is a molecule that causes vasodilation of your blood vessels, which means that more blood can reach your muscle tissue. As a result, l-citrulline delays fatigue (so you can work out harder and longer), enhances nutrient delivery to your muscles, and reduces post-workout soreness (so you can train hard again sooner).[11-12] Also, since citrulline improves blood flow, it helps you with obtaining a skin-splitting pump. Not only will this give you a physiological boost during your workouts, but it also aids muscle growth. If you want to supplement with citrulline to support exercise performance and fitness progress, take 6 grams of the amino acid one hour before your workout.

Multivitamin: As we've covered in step three, getting enough vitamins and minerals is crucial for your figure and athletic performance. This is because many of these nutrients are involved in bodily functions related to body composition, such as supporting metabolism and fat oxidation. And while optimizing your diet can help with obtaining these nutrients, unfortunately, that's often not enough. For example, research on popular diets—including ones that are rich in nutrient-dense foods—shows that such eating styles are often deficient in certain micronutrients.[13] So, to make sure that you get your daily needs of vitamins and minerals, it's wise to supplement with a multivitamin. (This is especially beneficial if you're on a weight-loss diet, because your nutrient intake tends to be lower.)

Vitamin D: A vitamin D deficiency is prevalent, with 41.6 percent of US adults and one billion people worldwide having low serum levels of the vitamin.[14-15] Not only does such a deficiency impair health and well-being, but it also hampers fitness goals because vitamin D is involved in many bodily functions related to body composition, including metabolism, appetite, and hormone production. So, it will do your vigor and fitness goals good if you optimize your vitamin D levels. While it would be best to get your levels checked through a blood test, if you don't get a lot of bare-skin sun exposure, supplement with a

1,000 to 2,000 IU dose of vitamin D3 per day. That's enough to meet the needs of most people.

Magnesium: This nutrient, which is the fourth most abundant mineral in the human body, is not only crucial for your health and well-being but also for your body and workouts. For example, magnesium affects energy production, oxygen uptake, and electrolyte balance; it's also essential for optimal workout performance.[16] The problem? Up to 75 percent of Americans don't meet their magnesium needs, and we athletes are especially prone to being deficient in this mineral.[17-18] The latter is because sweating raises magnesium requirements.[16]

One of the main reasons why magnesium deficiencies are so common is that grains—the primary food source of most Americans—are a poor source of the mineral. Further, magnesium-rich sources such as leafy vegetables and nuts are eaten only sparingly by most people. However, even if you consume many magnesium-dense foods, you can still be deficient in the mineral. This is because the magnesium content of the soil has plummeted over the years due to poor agricultural practices. So we're getting less of the mineral through diet.

While a high-quality multivitamin can help you get more magnesium, it's often not enough because most companies underdose magnesium and use cheap, ineffective forms. So it's better to supplement with the mineral individually. Consuming a product containing 400 milligrams of magnesium citrate a day will do the trick.

That's all? Yes, this is all we recommend for most people to get a small edge toward reaching their fitness goals. Sure, there are other compounds that may be beneficial, but most supplements lack research and work only in specific scenarios. If you want to try a particular compound but you're not sure whether it's beneficial, an excellent resource to evaluate its effectiveness is www.examine.com. It's an independent resource that summarizes the results of the available scientific research on a wide range of supplements so that you can easily see whether a compound is proven to work or not. (We're in no way, shape, or form associated with examine.com—it's just an excellent resource to determine the validity of specific compounds.)

Key Takeaways

- Most supplements are useless when it comes to helping you build a body that performs well and has the aesthetics to match.
- That said, the following seven supplements may give you a slight edge for reaching your goals: whey protein, creatine, caffeine, citrulline, a multivitamin, vitamin D, and magnesium.
- While other available compounds may also be beneficial, nearly all products on the market don't live up to their marketing claims and often are even harmful to your health and well-being.

Closing Thoughts

Ancient scripture says: If you don't know where you're going, any road will take you there.

When it comes to nutrition goals, many people are easily distracted and wander aimlessly, like a lost child in the toy aisle at a Target superstore.

That doesn't have to be you anymore!

All you have to decide is what you want. Do you want to bulk up? Do you want to lean out?

Once you decide, take this book and make it work for you.

You've already put in the time by going from the foundational advice in the early chapters and continuing through the ensuing sections with their increased specificity.

Now that you have read through the book, use your newly acquired information. Make this book work for you.

State your nutritional goal, make a plan, and implement it, your way!

References

Step 1: Calories

1. Golay, A., Allaz, A. F., Morel, Y., De Tonnac, N., Tankova, S., and Reaven, G. (1996). Similar weight loss with low- or high-carbohydrate diets. *American Journal of Clinical Nutrition, 63*(2), 174–8.
2. Sargrad, K. R., Homko, C., Mozzoli, M., and Boden, G. (2005). Effect of high protein vs high carbohydrate intake on insulin sensitivity, body weight, hemoglobin A1c, and blood pressure in patients with type 2 diabetes mellitus. *Journal of the American Dietetic Association, 105*(4), 573–80.
3. Leibel, R. L., Hirsch, J., Appel, B. E., and Checani, G. C. (1992). Energy intake required to maintain body weight is not affected by wide variation in diet composition. *American Journal of Clinical Nutrition, 55*(2), 350–5.
4. Astrup, A., Meinert Larsen, T., and Harper, A. (2004). Atkins and other low-carbohydrate diets: hoax or an effective tool for weight loss? *Lancet, 364*(9437), 897–9.
5. Parker, B., Noakes, M., Luscombe, N., and Clifton, P. (2002). Effect of a high-protein, high-monounsaturated fat weight loss diet on glycemic control and lipid levels in type 2 diabetes. *Diabetes Care, 25*(3), 425–30.
6. Heilbronn, L. K., Noakes, M., and Clifton, P. M. (1999). Effect of energy restriction, weight loss, and diet composition on plasma lipids and glucose in patients with type 2 diabetes. *Diabetes Care, 22*(6), 889–95.
7. Noakes, M., Keogh, J. B., Foster, P. R., and Clifton, P. M. (2005). Effect of an energy-restricted, high-protein, low-fat diet relative to a conventional high-carbohydrate, low-fat diet on weight loss, body composition, nutritional status, and markers of cardiovascular health in obese women. *American Journal of Clinical Nutrition, 81*(6), 1298–306.

8. Keogh, J. B., Luscombe-Marsh, N. D., Noakes, M., Wittert, G. A., and Clifton, P. M. (2007). Long-term weight maintenance and cardiovascular risk factors are not different following weight loss on carbohydrate-restricted diets high in either monounsaturated fat or protein in obese hyperinsulinaemic men and women. *British Journal of Nutrition, 97*(2), 405–10.
9. Luscombe-Marsh, N. D., Noakes, M., Wittert, G. A., Keogh, J. B., Foster, P., and Clifton, P. M. (2005). Carbohydrate-restricted diets high in either monounsaturated fat or protein are equally effective at promoting fat loss and improving blood lipids. *American Journal of Clinical Nutrition, 81*(4), 762–72.
10. Boden, G., Sargrad, K., Homko, C., Mozzoli, M., and Stein, T. P. (2005). Effect of a low-carbohydrate diet on appetite, blood glucose levels, and insulin resistance in obese patients with type 2 diabetes. *Annals of Internal Medicine, 15;142*(6), 403–11.
11. Brinkworth, G. D., Noakes, M., Keogh, J. B., Luscombe, N. D., Wittert, G. A., and Clifton, P. M. (2004). Long-term effects of a high-protein, low-carbohydrate diet on weight control and cardiovascular risk markers in obese hyperinsulinemic subjects. *International Journal of Obesity and Related Metabolic Disorders, 28*(5), 661–70.
12. Farnsworth, E., Luscombe, N. D., Noakes, M., Wittert, G., Argyiou, E., and Clifton, P. M. (2003). Effect of a high-protein, energy-restricted diet on body composition, glycemic control, and lipid concentrations in overweight and obese hyperinsulinemic men and women. *American Journal of Clinical Nutrition, 78*(1), 31–9.
13. Thomson, R. L., Buckley, J. D., Noakes, M., Clifton, P. M., Norman, R. J., and Brinkworth, G. D. (2008). The effect of a hypocaloric diet with and without exercise training on body composition, cardiometabolic risk profile, and reproductive function in overweight and obese women with polycystic ovary syndrome. *The Journal of Clinical Endocrinology & Metabolism, 93*(9), 3373–80.
14. Golay, A., Allaz, A. F., Ybarra, J., Bianchi, P., Saraiva, S., Mensi, N.,… De Tonnac, N. (2000). Similar weight loss with low-energy food combining or balanced diets. *International Journal of Obesity and Related Metabolic Disorders, 24*(4), 492–6.

15. Strasser, B., Spreitzer, A., and Haber, P. (2007). Fat loss depends on energy deficit only, independently of the method for weight loss. *Annals of Nutrition and Metabolism, 51*(5), 428–32.
16. McLaughlin, T., Carter, S., Lamendola, C., Abbasi, F., Yee, G., Schaaf, P., ...Reaven, G. (2006). Effects of moderate variations in macronutrient composition on weight loss and reduction in cardiovascular disease risk in obese, insulin-resistant adults. *American Journal of Clinical Nutrition, 84*(4), 813–21.
17. Golay, A., Eigenheer, C., Morel, Y., Kujawski, P., Lehmann, T., and De Tonnac, N. (1996). Weight-loss with low or high carbohydrate diet? *International Journal of Obesity and Related Metabolic Disorders, 20*(12), 1067–72.
18. Bray, G. A., Smith, S. R., De Jonge, L., Xie, H., Rood, J., Martin, C. K., ...Redman, L. M. (2012). Effect of dietary protein content on weight gain, energy expenditure, and body composition during overeating: a randomized controlled trial. *JAMA, 4;307*(1), 47–55.
19. Joosen, A. M., and Westerp, K. R. (2006). Energy expenditure during overfeeding. *Nutrition and Metabolism, 3,* 25.
20. Joosen, A. M., Bakker, A. H., and Westerp, K. R. (2005). Metabolic efficiency and energy expenditure during short-term overfeeding. *Physiology and Behavior, 85*(5), 593–7.
21. Tremblay, A., Despres, J. P., Theriault, G., Fournier, G., and Bouchard, C. (1992). Overfeeding and energy expenditure in humans. *American Journal of Clinical Nutrition, 56*(5), 857–62.
22. He, J., Votruba, S., Pomeroy, J., Bonfiglio, S., and Krakoff, J. (2012). Measurement of ad libitum food intake, physical activity, and sedentary time in response to overfeeding. *PLOS One, 7*(5), 36225.
23. Diaz, E. Q., Prentice, A. M., Goldberg, G. R., Murgatroyd, P. R., and Coward, W. A. (1992). Metabolic response to experimental overfeeding in lean and overweight healthy volunteers. *American Journal of Clinical Nutrition, 56*(4), 641–55.
24. Horton, T. J., Drougas, H., Brachey, A., Reed, G. W., Peters, J. C., and Hill, J. O. (1995). Fat and carbohydrate overfeeding in humans: Different effects on energy storage. *American Journal of Clinical Nutrition, 62*(1), 19–29.

25. Tappy, L. (2004). Metabolic consequences of overfeeding in humans. *Current Opinion in Clinical Nutrition and Metabolic Care, 7*(6), 623–8.
26. Park, M. (2010, November 8). Twinkie diet helps nutrition professor lose 27 pounds. Retrieved from http://edition.cnn.com/2010/HEALTH/11/08/twinkie.diet.professor/index.html.
27. Mifflin, M. D., St Jeor, S. T., Hill, L. A., Scott, B. J., Daugherty, S. A., & Koh, Y. O. (1990). A new predictive equation for resting energy expenditure in healthy individuals. *American Journal of Clinical Nutrition, 51*(2), 241–7.
28. Hendrickson, S., and Mattes, R. (2007). Financial incentive for diet recall accuracy does not affect reported energy intake or number of under-reporters in a sample of overweight females. *Journal of the American Dietetic Association, 107*(1), 118–21.
29. Bedard, D., Shatenstein, B., and Nadon, S. (2004). Underreporting of energy intake from a self-administered food-frequency questionnaire completed by adults in Montreal. *Public Health Nutrition, 7*(5), 675–81.
30. Poslusna, K., Ruprich, J., De Vries, J. H., Jakubikova, M., and van't Veer, P. (2009). Misreporting of energy and micronutrient intake estimated by food records and 24 hour recalls, control and adjustment methods in practice. *British Journal of Nutrition, 101 Suppl. 2,* S73–85.
31. Champagne, C. M., Bray, G. A., Krutz, A. A., Monteiro, J. B., Tucker, E., Volaufova, J., and Delany, J. P. (2002). Energy intake and energy expenditure: a controlled study comparing dietitians and non-dietitians. *Journal of the American Dietetic Association, 102*(10), 1428–32.
32. Cook, A., Pryer, J., and Shetty, P. (2000). The problem of accuracy in dietary surveys. Analysis of the over 65 UK National Diet and Nutrition Survey. *Journal of Epidemiology and Community Health, 54*(8), 611–6.
33. Petre, A. (2016, December 7). Does Calorie Counting Work? A Critical Look. Retrieved from https://www.healthline.com/nutrition/does-calorie-counting-work.
34. Hartmann-Boyce, J., Johns, D. J., Jebb, S. A., and Aveyard, P. (2014). Effect of behavioural techniques and delivery mode on effectiveness of weight management: systematic review, meta-analysis and meta-regression. *Obesity Reviews, 15*(7), 598–609.

35. Burke, L. E., Wang, J., and Sevick, M. A. (2011). Self-monitoring in weight loss: a systematic review of the literature. *Journal of the American Dietetic Association, 111*(1), 92–102.

Step 2: Macros

1. Hall, W. L., Millward, D. J., Long, S. J., and Morgan, L. M. (2003). Casein and whey exert different effects on plasma amino acid profiles, gastrointestinal hormone secretion and appetite. *British Journal of Nutrition, 89*(2), 239–48.
2. Batterham, R. L., Heffron, H., Kapoor, S., Chivers, J. E., Chandarana, K., Herzog, H., ... Withers, D. J. (2006). Critical role for peptide YY in protein-mediated satiation and body-weight regulation. *Cell Metabolism, 4*(3), 223–33.
3. Hannon-Engel, S. (2012). Regulating satiety in bulimia nervosa: the role of cholecystokinin. *Perspectives in Psychiatric Care, 48*(1), 34–40.
4. Lejeune, M. P., Westerterp, K. R., Adam, T. C., Luscombe-Marsh, N. D., and Westerterp-Plantenga, M. S. (2006). Ghrelin and glucagon-like peptide 1 concentrations, 24-h satiety, and energy and substrate metabolism during a high-protein diet and measured in a respiration chamber. *American Journal of Clinical Nutrition, 83*(1), 89–94.
5. Blom, W. A., Lluch, A., Stafleu, A., Vinoy, S., Holst, J. J., Schaafsma, G., and Hendriks, H. F. (2006). Effect of a high-protein breakfast on the postprandial ghrelin response. *American Journal of Clinical Nutrition, 83*(2), 211–20.
6. Weigle, D. S., Breen, P. A., Matthys, C. C., Callahan, H. S., Meeuws, K. E., Burden, V. R., and Purnell, J. Q. (2005). A high-protein diet induces sustained reductions in appetite, ad libitum caloric intake, and body weight despite compensatory changes in diurnal plasma leptin and ghrelin concentrations. *American Journal of Clinical Nutrition, 82*(1), 41–8.
7. Mettler, S., Mitchell, N., and Tipton, K. D. (2010). Increased protein intake reduces lean body mass loss during weight loss in athletes. *Medicine and Science in Sports and Exercise, 42*(2), 326–37.
8. Schiaffino, S., Dyar, K. A., Ciciliot, S., Blaauw, B., and Sandri, M. (2013). Mechanisms regulating skeletal muscle growth and atrophy. *The FEBS Journal, 280*(17), 4294–314.

9. Morton, R. W., Murphy, K. T., McKellar, S. R., Schoenfeld, B. J., Henselmans, M., Helms, E., ... Phillips, S. M. (2018). A systematic review, meta-analysis and meta-regression of the effect of protein supplementation on resistance training-induced gains in muscle mass and strength in healthy adults. *British Journal of Sports Medicine, 52*(6), 376–84.
10. Phillips, S. M., and Van Loon, L. J. (2011). Dietary protein for athletes: from requirements to optimum adaptation. *Journal of Sports Sciences, 29*, 29–38.
11. Miller, S. L., and Wolfe, R. R. (1999). Physical exercise as a modulator of adaptation to low and high carbohydrate and low and high fat intakes. *European Journal of Clinical Nutrition, 53*(1), 112–9.
12. Hämäläinen, E. K., Adlercreutz, H., Puska, P., and Pietinen, P. (1983). Decrease of serum total and free testosterone during a low-fat high-fibre diet. *Journal of Steroid Biochemistry, 18*(3), 369–70.
13. Volek, J. S., Kraemer, W. J., Bush, J. A., Incledon, T., and Boetes, M. (1997). Testosterone and cortisol in relationship to dietary nutrients and resistance exercise. *Journal of Applied Physiology, 82*(1), 49–54.
14. Smith, R. G. (2009). From GH to Billy Ghrelin. *Cell Metabolism, 10*(2), 82–3.
15. Tsitouras, P. D., Gucciardo, F., Salbe, A. D., Heward, C., and Harman, S. M. (2008). High omega-3 fat intake improves insulin sensitivity and reduces CRP and IL6, but does not affect other endocrine axes in healthy older adults. *Hormone and Metabolic Research, 40*(3), 199–205.
16. Paolisso, G., Tagliamonte, M. R., Rizzo, M. R., and Giugliano, D. (1999). Advancing age and insulin resistance: new facts about an ancient history. *European Journal of Clinical Investigation, 29*(9), 758–69.
17. Danadian, K., Balasekaran, G., Lewy, V., Meza, M. P., Robertson, R., and Arslanian, S. A. (1999). Insulin sensitivity in African-American children with and without family history of type 2 diabetes. *Diabetes Care, 22*(8), 1325–9.
18. Arslanian, S. A., Bacha, F., Saad, R., and Gungor, N. (2005). Family history of type 2 diabetes is associated with decreased insulin sensitivity and an impaired balance between insulin sensitivity and insulin secretion in white youth. *Diabetes Care, 28*(1), 115–9.

19. Svendsen, P. F., Nilas, L., Norgaard, K., Jensen, J. E., and Madsbad, S. (2008). Obesity, body composition and metabolic disturbances in polycystic ovary syndrome. *Human Reproduction, 23*(9), 2113–21.
20. Awdishu, S., Williams, N. I., Laredo, S. E., and De Souza, M. J. (2009). Oligomenorrhoea in exercising women: a polycystic ovarian syndrome phenotype or distinct entity? *Sports Medicine, 39*(12), 1055–69.
21. Siler, S. Q., Neese, R. A., and Hellerstein, M. K. (1999). De novo lipogenesis, lipid kinetics, and whole-body lipid balances in humans after acute alcohol consumption. *American Journal of Clinical Nutrition, 70*(5), 928–36.
22. Preedy, V. R., Reilly, M. E., Patel, V. B., Richardson, P. J., and Peters, T. J. (n.d.). Protein metabolism in alcoholism: effects on specific tissues and the whole body. *Nutrition, 15*(7–8), 604–8.

Step 3: Food Selection

1. Duncan, K. H., Bacon, J. A., and Weinsier, R. L. (1983). The effects of high and low energy density diets on satiety, energy intake, and eating time of obese and nonobese subjects. *American Journal of Clinical Nutrition, 37*(5), 763–7.
2. Holt, S. H., Miller, J. C., Petocz, P., and Farmakalidis, E. (1995). A satiety index of common foods. *European Journal of Clinical Nutrition, 49*(9), 675–90.
3. Jalali, G. R., Roozbeh, J., Mohammadzadeh, A., Sharifian, M., Sagheb, M. M., Hamidian Jahromi, A., …Afshariani, R. (2010). Impact of oral zinc therapy on the level of sex hormones in male patients on hemodialysis. *Renal Failure, 32*(4), 417–8.
4. Maxwell, C., and Volpe, S. L. (2007). Effect of zinc supplementation on thyroid hormone function. A case study of two college females. *Annals of Nutrition and Metabolism, 51*(2), 188–94.
5. Wishnofsky, M. (1958). Caloric equivalents of gained or lost weight. *American Journal of Clinical Nutrition, 6*(5), 542–6.

Step 4: Meal Frequency

1. Cameron, J. D., Cyr, M. J., and Doucet, E. (2010). Increased meal frequency does not promote greater weight loss in subjects who were

prescribed an 8-week equi-energetic energy-restricted diet. *British Journal of Nutrition, 103*(8), 1098–101.
2. Verboeket-van de Venne, W. P., and Westerp, K. R. (1993). Frequency of feeding, weight reduction and energy metabolism. *International Journal of Obesity and Related Metabolic Disorders, 17*(1), 31–6.
3. Bellisle, F., McDevitt, R., and Prentice, A. M. (1997). Meal frequency and energy balance. *British Journal of Nutrition, 77*(1), 57–70.
4. Helms, E. R., Aragon, A. A., and Fitschen, P. J. (2014). Evidence-based recommendations for natural bodybuilding contest preparation: nutrition and supplementation. *Journal of the International Society of Sports Nutrition, 12,* 11–20.
5. Henselmans, M. (n.d.). Do you need 4 meals per day for maximum growth after all? Retrieved from https://bayesianbodybuilding.com/meal-frequency-science/.
6. Farshchi, H. R., Taylor, M. A., and Macdonald, I. A. (2004). Decreased thermic effect of food after an irregular compared with a regular meal pattern in healthy lean women. *International Journal of Obesity and Related Metabolic Disorders, 28*(5), 653–60.
7. Farshchi, H. R., Taylor, M. A., and Macdonald, I. A. (2004). Regular meal frequency creates more appropriate insulin sensitivity and lipid profiles compared with irregular meal frequency in healthy lean women. *European Journal of Clinical Nutrition, 58*(7), 1071–7.

Step 5: Nutrient Timing

1. Helms, E. R., Aragon, A. A., and Fitschen, P. J. (2014). Evidence-based recommendations for natural bodybuilding contest preparation: nutrition and supplementation. *Journal of the International Society of Sports Nutrition, 12,* 11–20.
2. Schoenfeld, B. J., Aragon, A. A., and Krieger, J. W. (2013). The effect of protein timing on muscle strength and hypertrophy: a meta-analysis. *Journal of the International Society of Sports Nutrition, 10*(1), 53.
3. Surina, D. M., Langhans, W., Pauli, R., and Wenk, C. (1993). Meal composition affects postprandial fatty acid oxidation. *American Journal of Physiology, 264*(6 pt 2), R1065–70.

4. Hargreaves, M., Hawley, J. A., and Jeukendrup, A. (2004). Pre-exercise carbohydrate and fat ingestion: effects on metabolism and performance. *Journal of Sports Sciences, 22*(1), 31–8.
5. Tsintzas, K., Williams, C., Constantin-Teodosiu, D., Hultman, E., Boobis, L., and Greenhaff, P. (2000). Carbohydrate ingestion prior to exercise augments the exercise-induced activation of the pyruvate dehydrogenase complex in human skeletal muscle. *Experimental Physiology, 85*(5), 581–6.
6. Miller, S. L., and Wolfe, R. R. (1999). Physical exercise as a modulator of adaptation to low and high carbohydrate and low and high fat intakes. *European Journal of Clinical Nutrition, 53*(1), 112–9.
7. Henselmans, M. (n.d.). Post-workout carbs: Are you drinking tons of sugar for no reason? Retrieved from https://bayesianbodybuilding.com/optimized-workout-nutrition-carbs-protein-revisited/.
8. Groen, B. B., Res, P. T., Pennings, B., Hertle, E., Senden, J. M., Saris, W. H., and Van Loon, L. J. (2012). Intragastric protein administration stimulates overnight muscle protein synthesis in elderly men. *American Journal of Physiology: Endocrinology and Metabolism, 1;302*(1), 52–60.
9. Res, P. T., Groen, B., Pennings, B., Beelen, M., Wallis, G. A., Gijsen, A. P., …Van Loon, J. L. (2012). Protein ingestion before sleep improves postexercise overnight recovery. *Medicine and Science in Sports and Exercise, 44*(8), 1560–9.
10. Afaghi, A., O'Connor, H., and Chow, C. M. (2007). High-glycemic-index carbohydrate meals shorten sleep onset. *American Journal of Clinical Nutrition, 85*(2), 426–30.
11. Gelfand, R. A., and Barrett, E. J. (1987). Effect of physiologic hyperinsulinemia on skeletal muscle protein synthesis and breakdown in man. *Journal of Clinical Investigation, 80*(1), 1–6.
12. Gonzalez, J. T., Veasey, R. C., Rumbold, P. L., and Stevenson, E. J. (2013). Breakfast and exercise contingently affect postprandial metabolism and energy balance in physically active males. *British Journal of Nutrition, 110*(4), 721–32.
13. Levitsky, D. A., and Pacanowski, C. R. (2013). Effect of skipping breakfast on subsequent energy intake. *Physiology and Behavior, 2*(119), 9–16.

14. Geliebter, A., Astbury, N. M., Aviram-Friedman, R., Yahav, E., and Hashim, S. (2014). Skipping breakfast leads to weight loss but also elevated cholesterol compared with consuming daily breakfasts of oat porridge or frosted cornflakes in overweight individuals: a randomised controlled trial. *Journal of Nutritional Sciences, 13*(3), 56.
15. LeCheminant, G. M., LeCheminant, J. D., Tucker, L. A., and Bailey, B. W. (2017). A randomized controlled trial to study the effects of breakfast on energy intake, physical activity, and body fat in women who are nonhabitual breakfast eaters. *Appetite, 1*(112), 44–51.

Step 6: Hydration

1. Yoon, C. K. (1998, June 16). U.S. Drinking Itself Dry, Study Finds. Retrieved from https://www.nytimes.com/1998/06/16/science/us-drinking-itself-dry-study-finds.html.
2. Popkin, B. M., Barclay, D. V., and Nielsen, S. J. (2005). Water and food consumption patterns of U.S. adults from 1999 to 2001. *Obesity Research, 13*(12), 2146–52.
3. Wishnofsky, M. (1958). Caloric equivalents of gained or lost weight. *American Journal of Clinical Nutrition, 6*(5), 542–6.
4. Kraft, J. A., Green, J. M., Bischop, P. A., Richardson, M. T., Neggers, Y. H., and Leeper, J. D. (2010). Impact of dehydration on a full body resistance exercise protocol. *European Journal of Applied Physiology, 109*(2), 259–67.
5. Adams, W. M., and Casa, D. J. (n.d.). The Influence of Hydration on Strength. Retrieved from https://ksi.uconn.edu/wp-content/uploads/sites/1222/2015/04/Strength-and-Hydration.pdf.
6. Popkin, B. M., D'Anci, K. E., and Rosenberg, I. H. (2010). Water, hydration and health. *Nutrition Reviews, 68*(8), 439–58.
7. Keller, U., Szinnai, G., Bilz, S., and Berneis, K. (2003). Effects of changes in hydration on protein, glucose and lipid metabolism in man: impact on health. *European Journal of Clinical Nutrition, 57*(2), 69–74.
8. Davy, B. M., Dennis, E. A., Dengo, A. L., Wilson, K. L., and Davy, K. P. (2008). Water consumption reduces energy intake at a breakfast meal in obese older adults. *Journal of the American Dietetic Association, 108*(7), 1236–9.

Step 7: Diet Breaks and Refeeds

1. Rosenbaum, M., Hirsch, J., Gallagher, D. A., and Leibel, R. L. (2008). Long-term persistence of adaptive thermogenesis in subjects who have maintained a reduced body weight. *American Journal of Clinical Nutrition, 88*(4), 906–12.
2. Joosen, A. M., and Westerterp, K. R. (2006). Energy expenditure during overfeeding. *Nutrition and Metabolism, 3,* 25.
3. Pratley, R. E., Nicolson, M., Bogardus, C., and Ravussin, E. (1997). Plasma leptin responses to fasting in Pima Indians. *American Journal of Physiology, 273*(3 pt 1), 644–9.
4. Davis, J. F. (2010). Adipostatic regulation of motivation and emotion. *Discovery Medicine, 9*(48), 462–7.
5. Davis, J. F., Choi, D. L., and Benoit, S. C. (2010). Insulin, leptin and reward. *Trends Endocrinology Metabolism, 21*(2), 68–74.
6. Forbes, G. B., Brown, M. R., Welle, S. L., and Underwood, L. E. (1989). Hormonal response to overfeeding. *American Journal of Clinical Nutrition, 49*(4), 608–11.
7. Dirlewanger, M., Di Vetta, V., Guenat, E., Battilana, P., Seematter, G., Schneiter, P., ... Tappy, L. (2000). Effects of short-term carbohydrate or fat overfeeding on energy expenditure and plasma leptin concentrations in healthy female subjects. *International Journal of Obesity and Related Metabolic Disorders, 24*(11), 1413–8.
8. Byrne, N. M., Sainsbury, A., King, N. A., Hills, A. P., and Wood, R. E. (2018). Intermittent energy restriction improves weight loss efficiency in obese men: the MATADOR study. *International Journal of Obesity, 42*(2), 129–38.
9. Dirlewanger, M., Di Vetta, V., Guenat, E., Battilana, P., Seematter, G., Schneiter, P., ... Tappy, L. (2000). Effects of short-term carbohydrate or fat overfeeding on energy expenditure and plasma leptin concentrations in healthy female subjects. *International Journal of Obesity and Related Metabolic Disorders, 24*(11), 1413–8.
10. Kreitzman, S. N., Coxon, A. Y., and Szaz, K. F. (1992). Glycogen storage: illusions of easy weight loss, excessive weight regain, and distortions in estimates of body composition. *American Journal of Clinical Nutrition, 56*(1), 292–3.

11. Dirlewanger, M., Di Vetta, V., Guenat, E., Battilana, P., Seematter, G., Schneiter, P., ...Tappy, L. (2000). Effects of short-term carbohydrate or fat overfeeding on energy expenditure and plasma leptin concentrations in healthy female subjects. *International Journal of Obesity and Related Metabolic Disorders, 24*(11), 1413–8.
12. Kreitzman, S. N., Coxon, A. Y., and Szaz, K. F. (1992). Glycogen storage: illusions of easy weight loss, excessive weight regain, and distortions in estimates of body composition. *American Journal of Clinical Nutrition, 56*(1), 292–3.

Step 8: Supplements

1. Campbell, B., Kreider, R. B., Ziegenfuss, T., La Bounty, P., Roberts, M., Burke, D., ...Antonio, J. (2007). International Society of Sports Nutrition position stand: protein and exercise. *Journal of the International Society of Sports Nutrition, 26,* 4–8.
2. Rawson, E. S., and Volek, J. S. (2003). Effects of creatine supplementation and resistance training on muscle strength and weightlifting performance. *Journal of Strength and Conditioning Research, 17*(4), 822–31.
3. Nissen, S. L., and Sharp, R. L. (2003). Effect of dietary supplements on lean mass and strength gains with resistance exercise: a meta-analysis. *Journal of Applied Physiology, 94*(2), 651–9.
4. Persky, A. M., and Brazeau, G. A. (2001). Clinical pharmacology of the dietary supplement creatine monohydrate. *Pharmacological Reviews, 53*(2), 161–76.
5. Del Coso, J., Salinero, J. J., González-Millán, C., Abián-Vicén, J., and Pérez-González, P. (2012). Dose response effects of a caffeine-containing energy drink on muscle performance: a repeated measures design. *Journal of the International Society of Sports Nutrition, 8;9*(1), 21.
6. Glaister, M., Howatson, G., Abraham, C. S., Lockey, R. A., Goodwin, J. E., Foley, P., and McInnes, G. (2008). Caffeine supplementation and multiple sprint running performance. *Medicine and Science in Sports and Exercise, 40*(10), 1835–40.
7. Ganio, M. S., Johnson, E. C., Klau, J. F., Anderson, J. M., Casa, D. J., Maresh, C. M., ...Armstrong, L. E. (2011). Effect of ambient temperature

on caffeine ergogenicity during endurance exercise. *European Journal of Applied Physiology, 111*(6), 1135–46.
8. Schneiker, K. T., Bishop, D., Dawson, B., and Hacklett, L. P. (2006). Effects of caffeine on prolonged intermittent-sprint ability in team-sport athletes. *Medicine and Science in Sports and Exercise, 38*(3), 578–85.
9. Carr, A. J., Gore, C. J., and Dawson, B. (2011). Induced alkalosis and caffeine supplementation: effects on 2,000-m rowing performance. *International Journal of Sport Nutrition and Exercise Metabolism, 21*(5), 357–64.
10. Sureda, A., Cordova, A., Ferrer, M. D., Pérez, G., Tur, J. A., and Pons, A. (2010). L-citrulline-malate influence over branched chain amino acid utilization during exercise. *European Journal of Applied Physiology, 110*(2), 341–51.
11. Wax, B., Kavazis, A. N., Weldon, K., and Sperlak, J. (2015). Effects of supplemental citrulline malate ingestion during repeated bouts of lower-body exercise in advanced weightlifters. *The Journal of Strength and Conditioning Research, 29*(3), 786–92.
12. Pérez-Guisado, J., and Jakerman, P. M. (2010). Citrulline malate enhances athletic anaerobic performance and relieves muscle soreness. *The Journal of Strength and Conditioning Research, 24*(5), 1215–22.
13. Calton, J. B. (2010). Prevalence of micronutrient deficiency in popular diet plans. *Journal of the International Society of Sports Nutrition, 7,* 24.
14. Forrest, K. Y., and Stuhldreher, W. L. (2011). Prevalence and correlates of vitamin D deficiency in US adults. *Nutrition Research, 31*(1), 48–54.
15. Sahota, O. (2014). Understanding vitamin D deficiency. *Age and Ageing, 43*(5), 589–91.
16. Nielsen, F. H., and Lukaski, H. C. (2006). Update on the relationship between magnesium and exercise. *Magnesium Research, 19*(3), 180–9.
17. Guerrera, M. P., Volpe, S. L., and Mao, J. J. (2009). Therapeutic uses of magnesium. *American Family Physician, 80*(2), 157–62.
18. Helms, E. R., Aragon, A. A., and Fitschen, P. J. (2014). Evidence-based recommendations for natural bodybuilding contest preparation: nutrition and supplementation. *Journal of the International Society of Sports Nutrition, 12,* 11–20.
19. Nielsen, F. H., and Lukaski, H. C. (2006). Update on the relationship between magnesium and exercise. *Magnesium Research, 19*(3), 180–9.

Made in the USA
Coppell, TX
18 September 2020